I0801210

MY FRIEND WITH HEALTH NEEDS

MY FRIEND WITH DIABETES

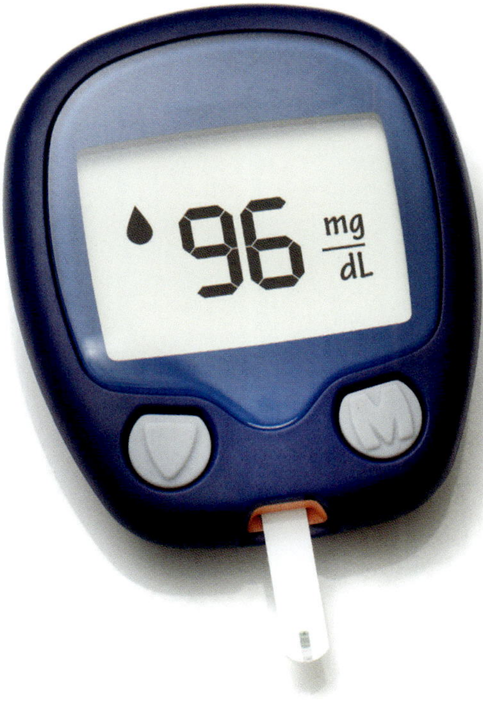

by Elizabeth Andrews

Cody Koala
An Imprint of Pop!
popbooksonline.com

Hello! My name is Cody Koala

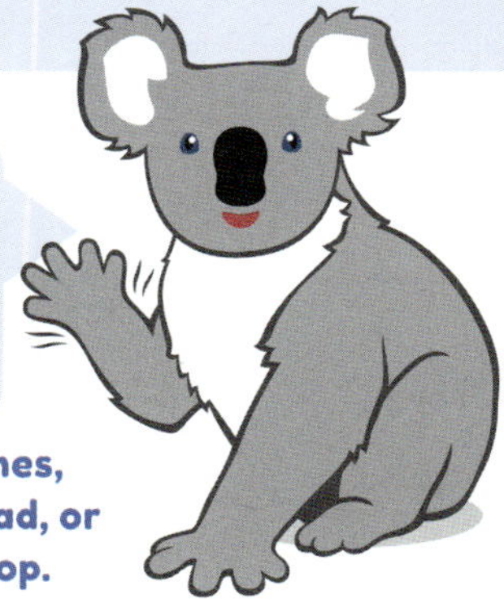

This book is filled with videos, puzzles, games, and more! Scan the QR codes* while you read, or visit the website below to make this book pop.

popbooksonline.com/diabetes

*Scanning QR codes requires a web-enabled smart device with a QR code reader app and a camera.

abdobooks.com
Published by Pop!, a division of ABDO, PO Box 398166, Minneapolis, Minnesota 55439. Copyright ©2024 by Abdo Consulting Group, Inc. International copyrights reserved in all countries. No part of this book may be reproduced in any form without written permission from the publisher. Cody Koala™ is a trademark and logo of Pop!.

Printed in the United States of America, North Mankato, Minnesota.
102023
012024

THIS BOOK CONTAINS RECYCLED MATERIALS

Cover Photo: Shutterstock Images
Interior Photos: Shutterstock Images; Getty Images
Editor: Grace Hansen
Series Designer: Victoria Bates

Library of Congress Control Number: 2023938825

Publisher's Cataloging-in-Publication Data
Names: Andrews, Elizabeth, author.
Title: My friend with diabetes / by Elizabeth Andrews
Description: Minneapolis, Minnesota : Pop!, 2024 | Series: My friend with health needs | Includes online resources and index
Identifiers: ISBN 9781098245313 (lib. bdg.) | ISBN 9781098245870 (ebook)
Subjects: LCSH: Friendship--Juvenile literature. | Diabetes--Juvenile literature. | Diabetes in children--Juvenile literature. | Social acceptance--Juvenile literature.
Classification: DDC 616.462--dc23

Table of Contents

Chapter 1

Type 1 Diabetes

Ian's friend Mason is sleeping over. Mason notices a white device on Ian's arm. "What is that?" Mason asks. Ian explains that it is a **blood sugar** monitor. It helps Ian. Ian has type 1 diabetes.

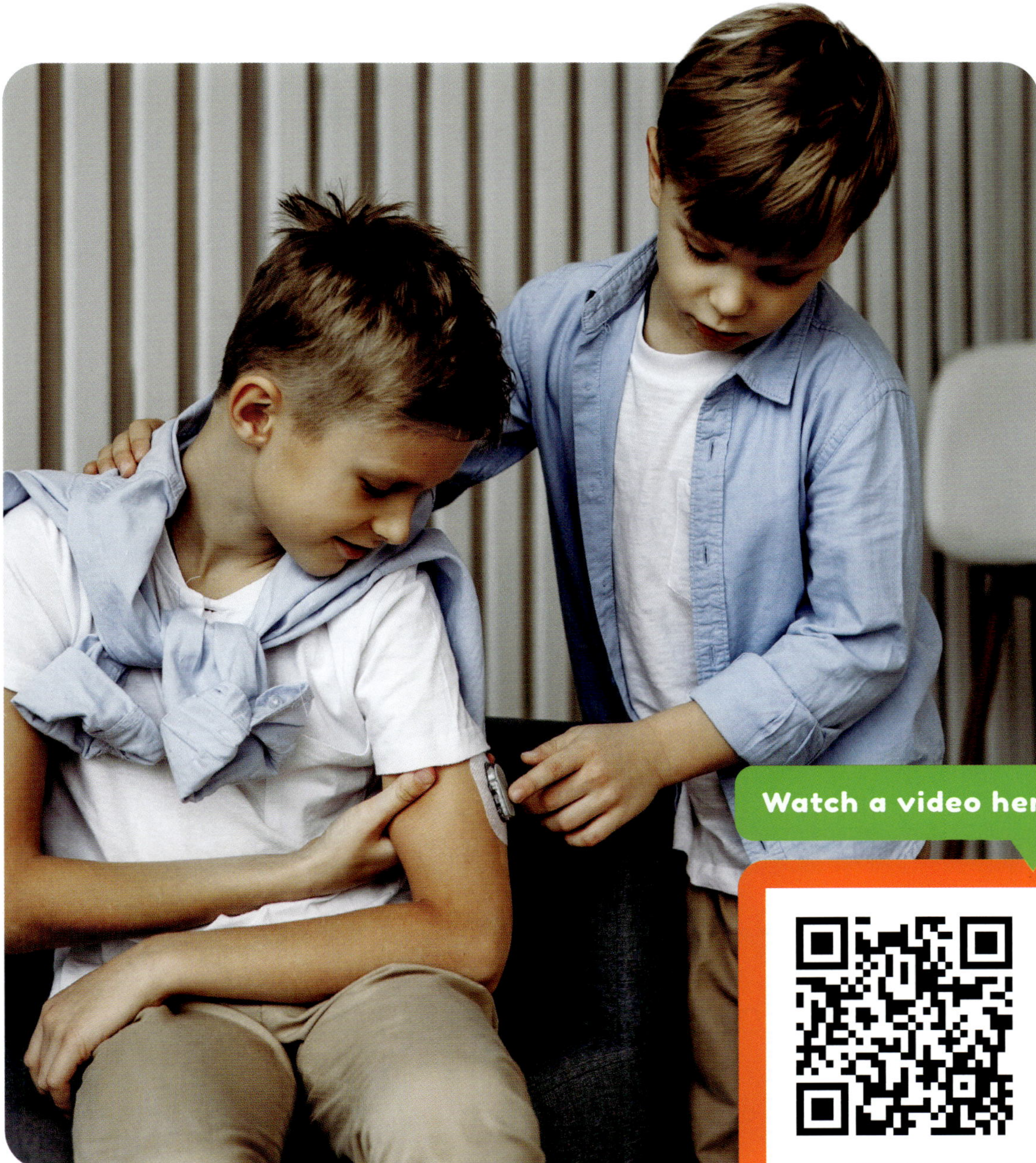

Watch a video here!

Chapter 2

What Is Diabetes?

Diabetes affects how the body uses and stores sugar. Usually, a **hormone** called **insulin** tells the body to what to do with sugar. But people with diabetes make little to no insulin.

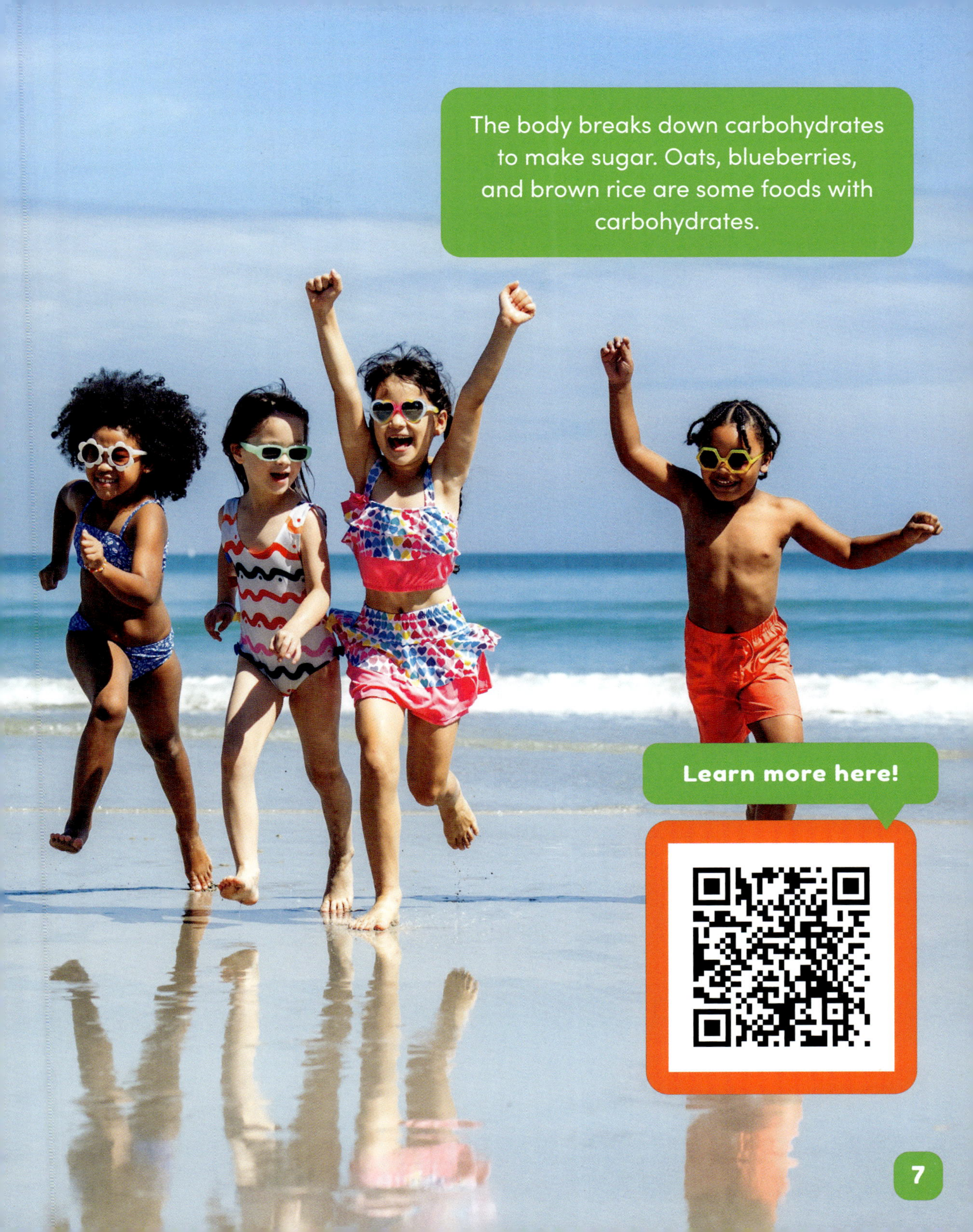

The body breaks down carbohydrates to make sugar. Oats, blueberries, and brown rice are some foods with carbohydrates.

Learn more here!

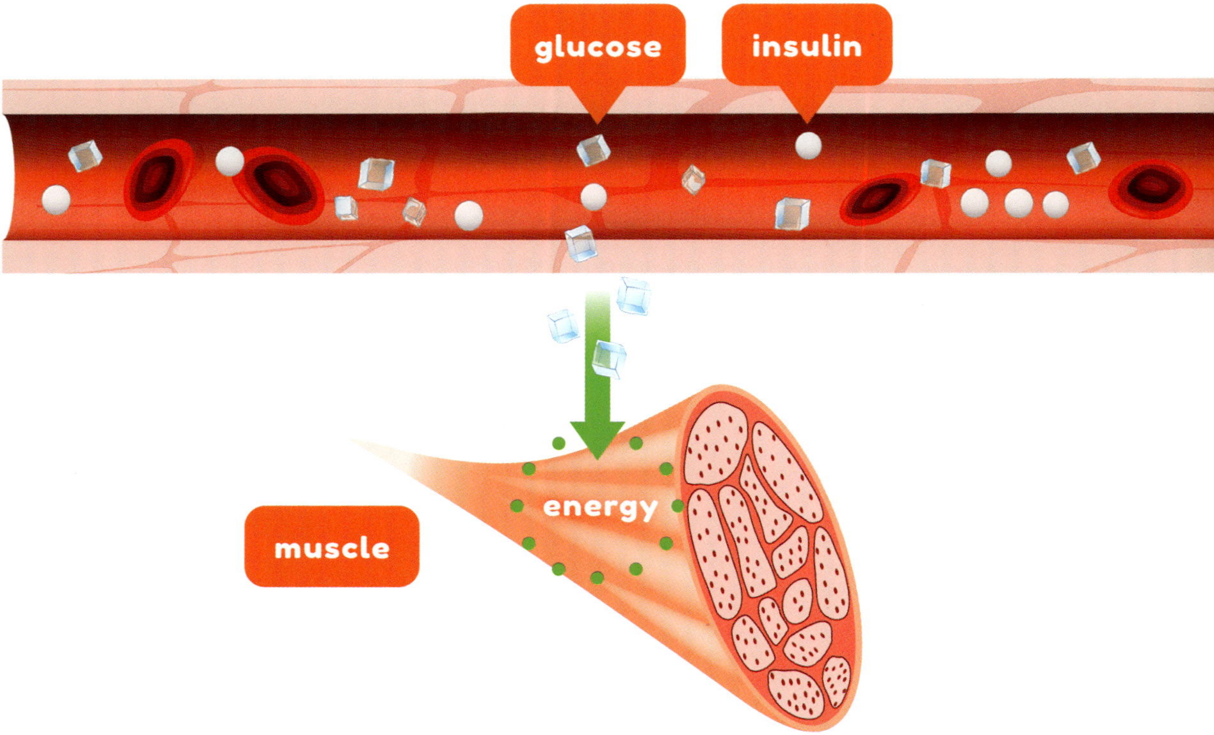

When a person without diabetes eats, their body breaks down their food into a sugar called glucose.

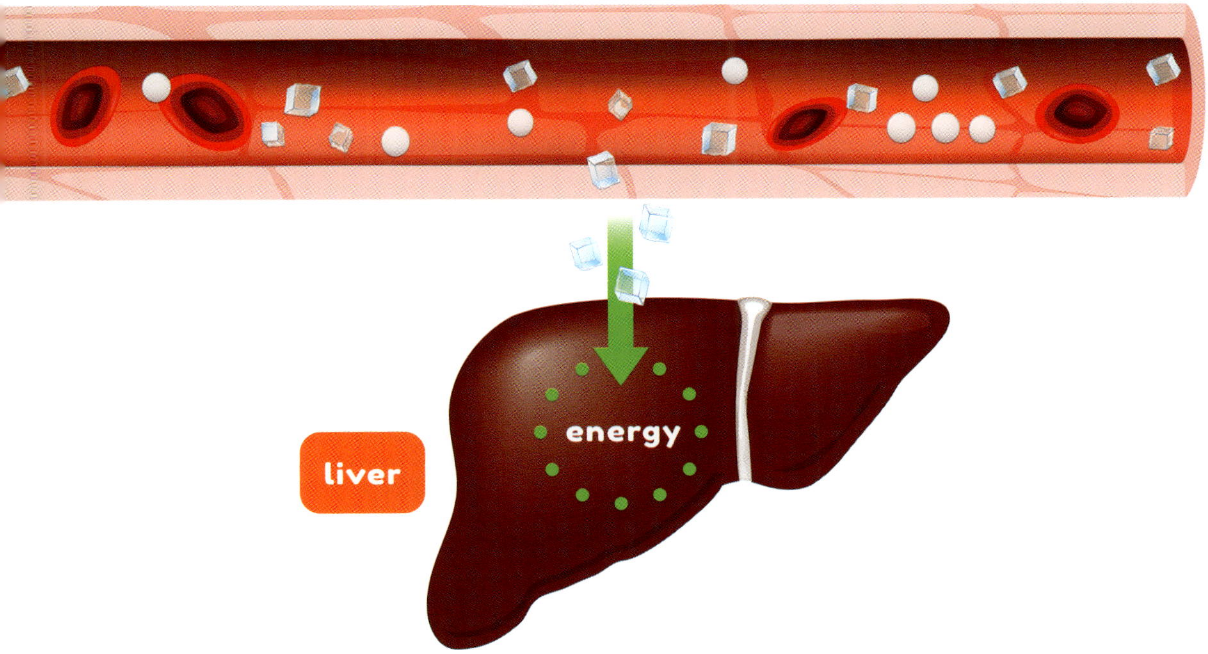

When glucose enters the blood, the body releases insulin. Insulin helps glucose enter the body's cells to give them energy.

Chapter 3

Caring for Diabetes

Glucose is not made into energy in a person with diabetes. Instead, it stays in the blood. This is hard on the body. People with diabetes pay attention to their **blood sugar** levels and take **insulin**.

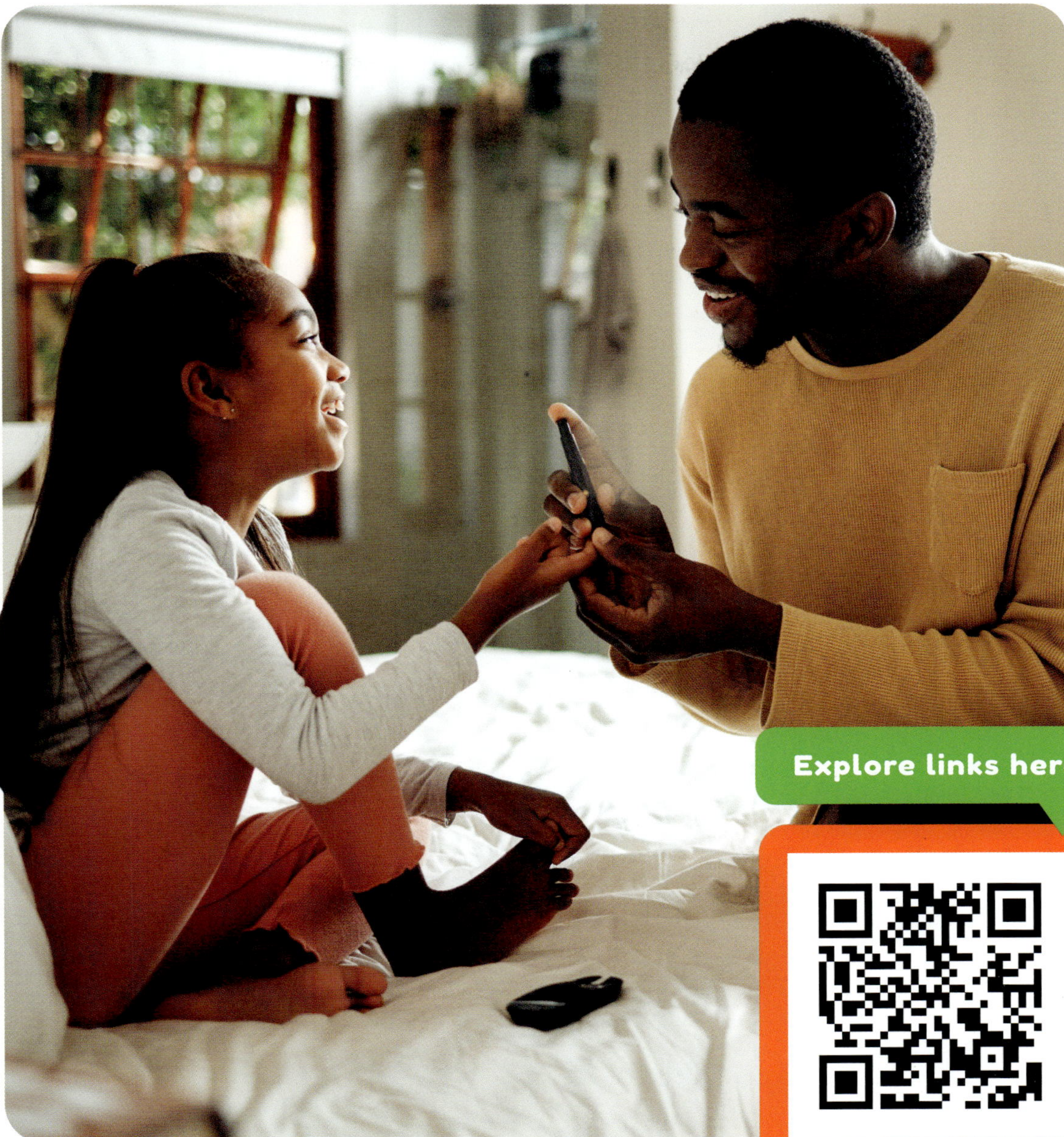

Explore links here!

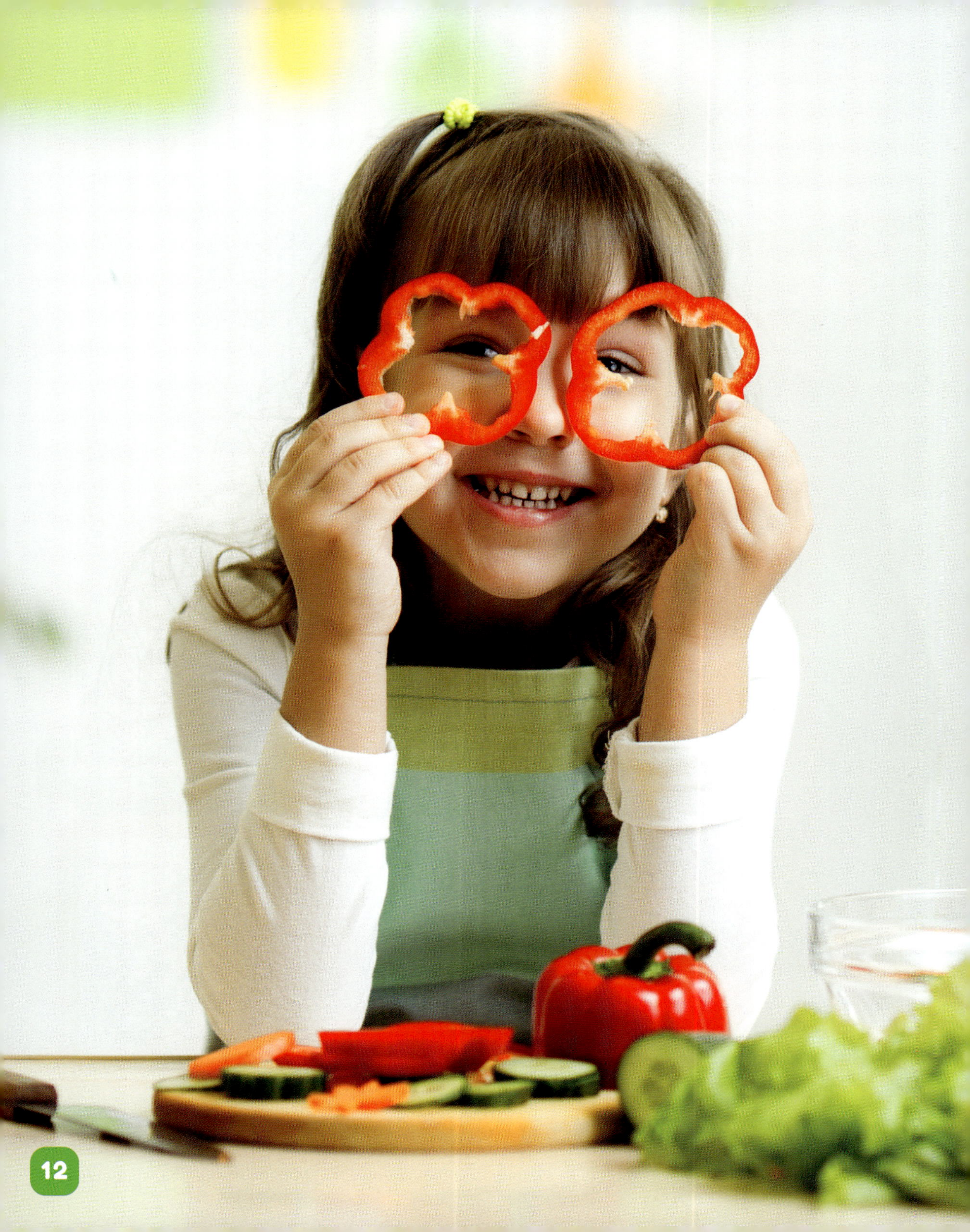

People with diabetes test their blood sugar levels often. They check levels before eating, before bed, before exercising, and whenever they feel like they have low or high blood sugar.

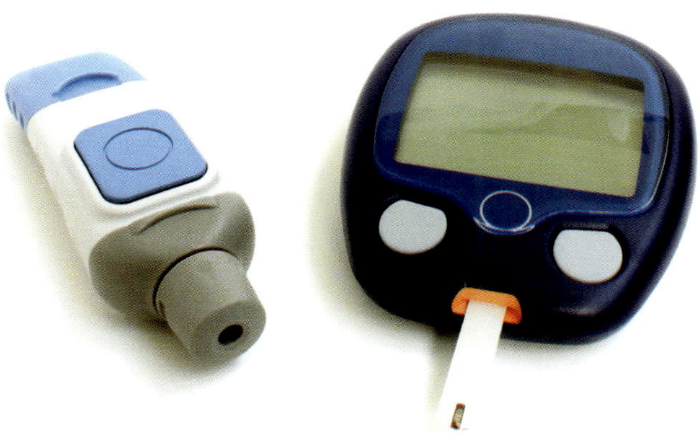

When a person has high blood sugar, they may use the bathroom a lot and have a stomach ache. They might also feel tired, thirsty, and **irritable**. Taking insulin fixes this.

Blood sugar that is too low or high can become life threatening.

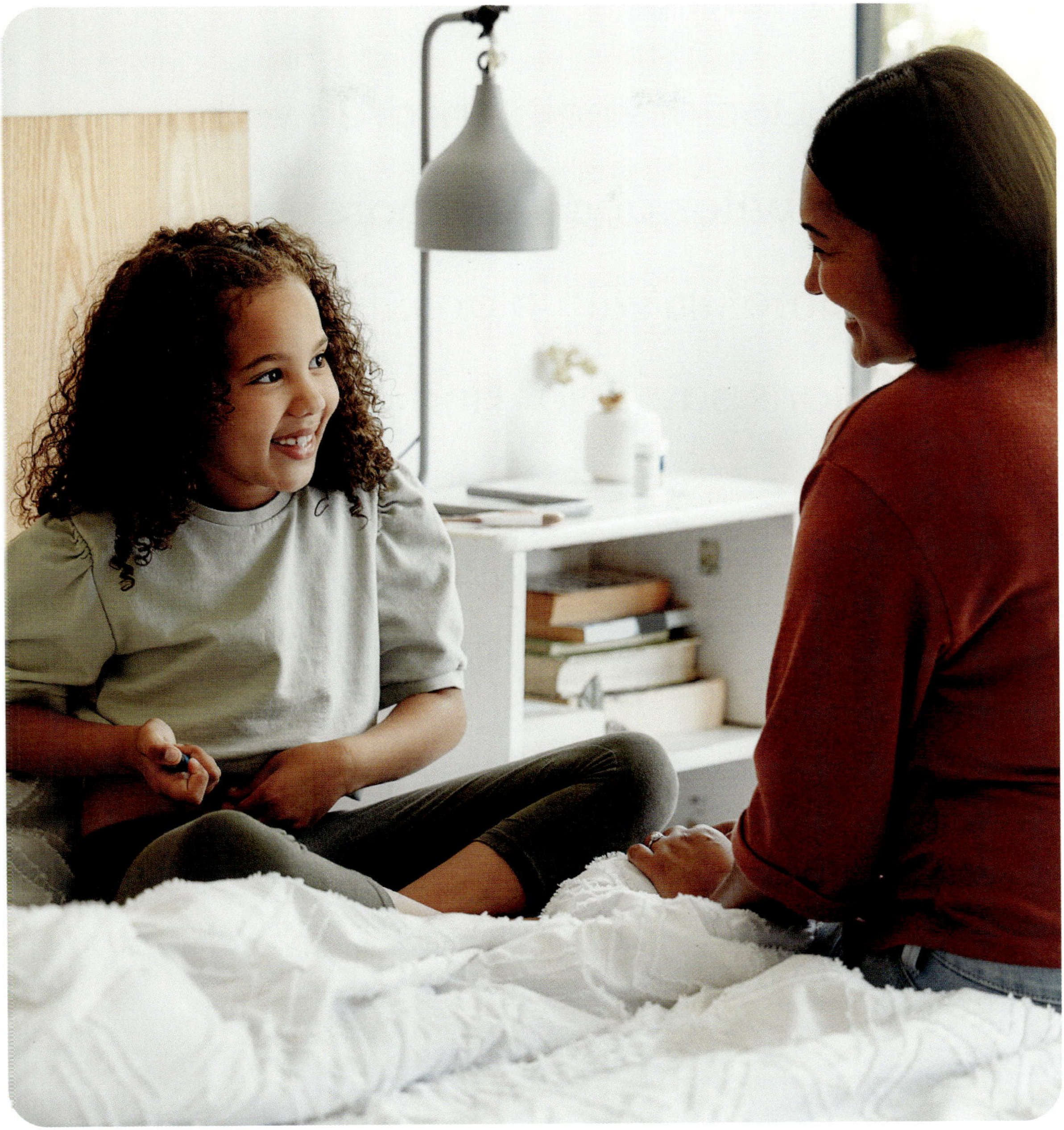

Doctors help children with diabetes and their parents come up with plans. These plans say what kind of insulin

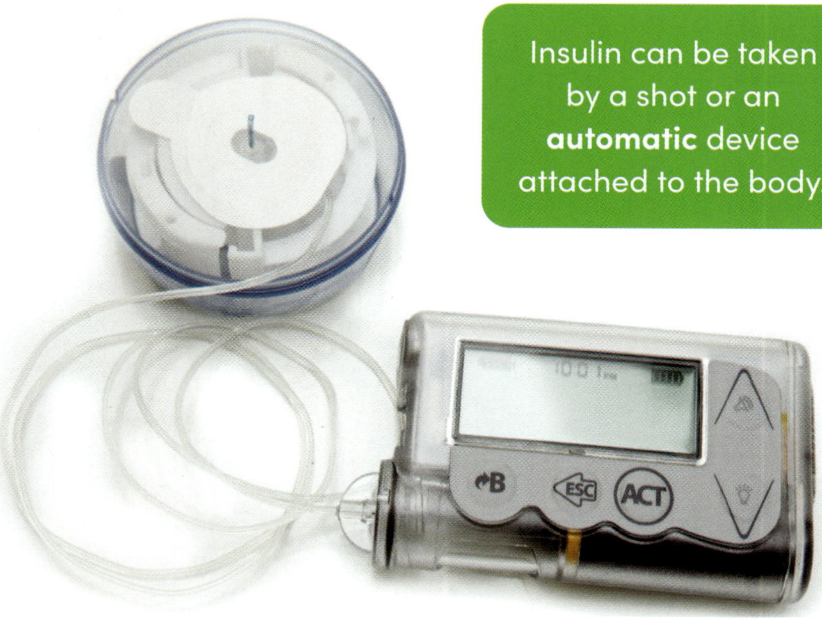

Insulin can be taken by a shot or an **automatic** device attached to the body.

to take and when to take it. Usually, insulin is taken before meals to control blood sugar.

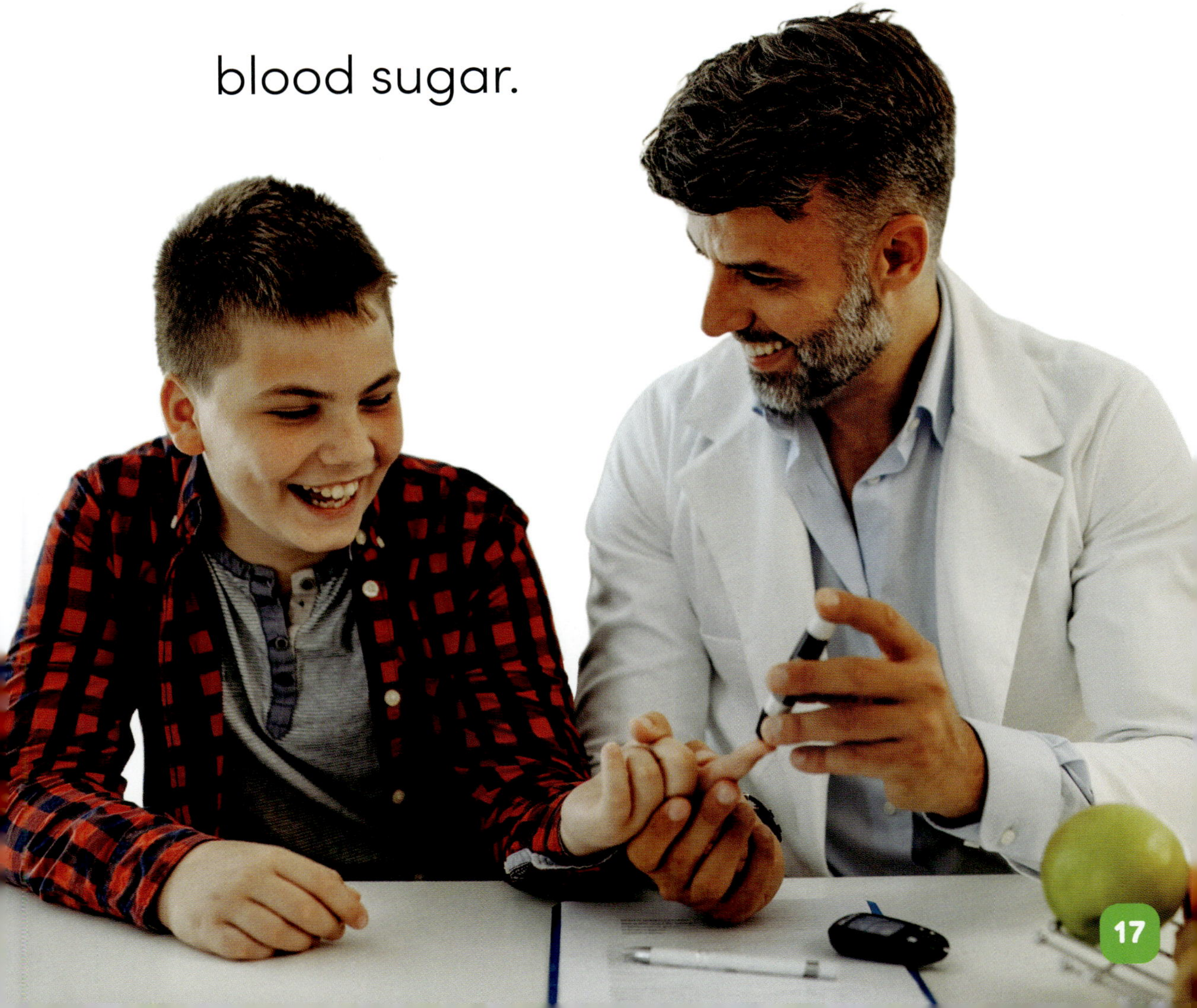

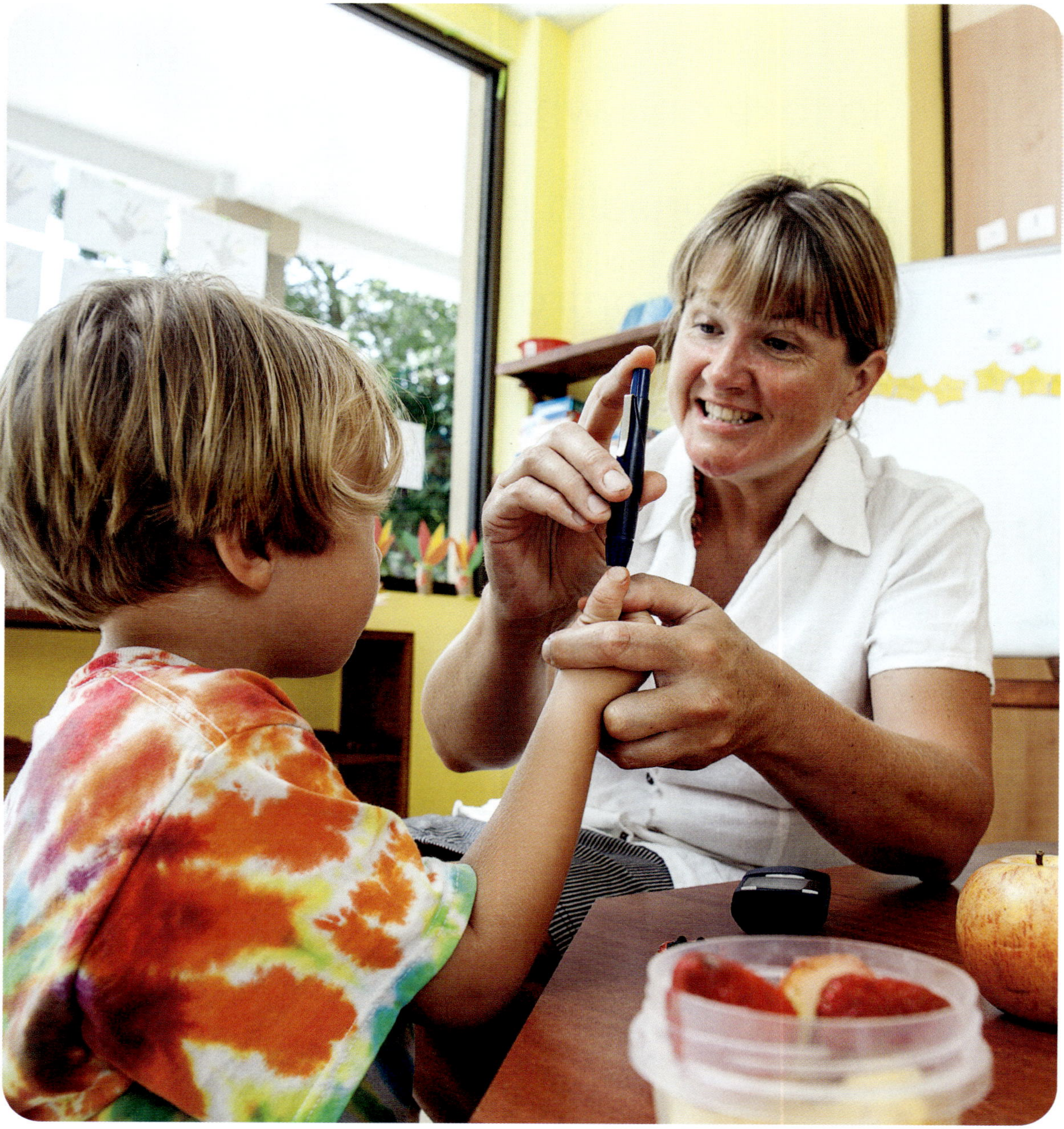

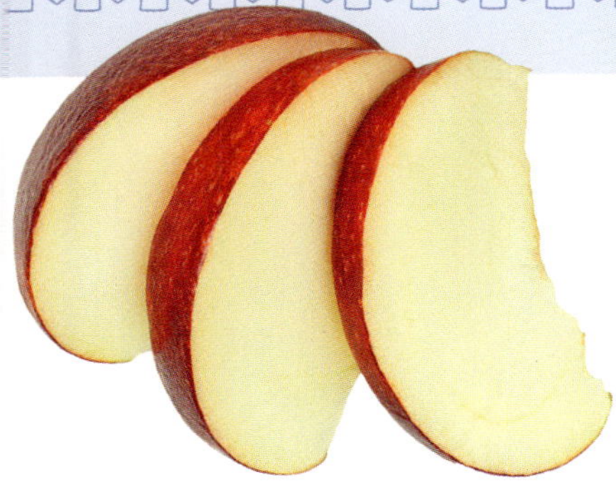

If a classmate starts to feel that their blood sugar is off, they will go to the school nurse. The nurse can help them check their levels. If their blood sugar is low, they have a snack. If it is high, they take insulin.

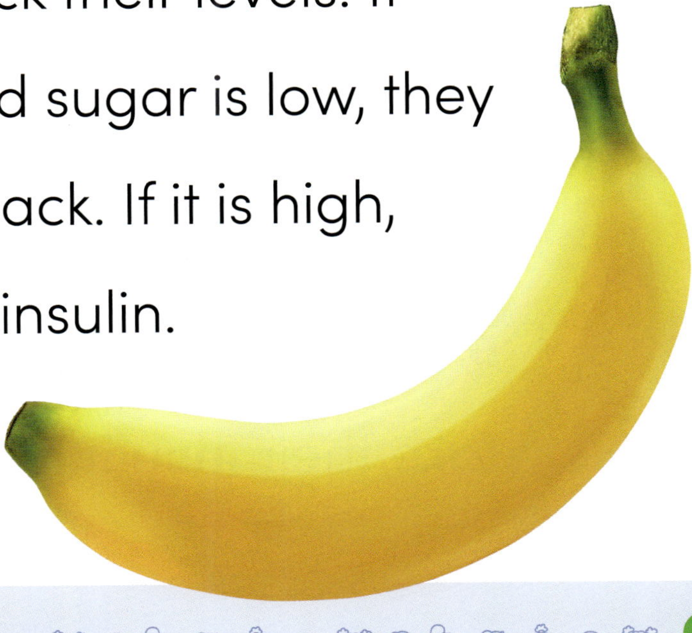

Chapter 4

Your Friend with Diabetes

Often, children with diabetes can enjoy life just like their friends! It's just more important for them to eat the right foods, get good exercise, and remember to take their **insulin**.

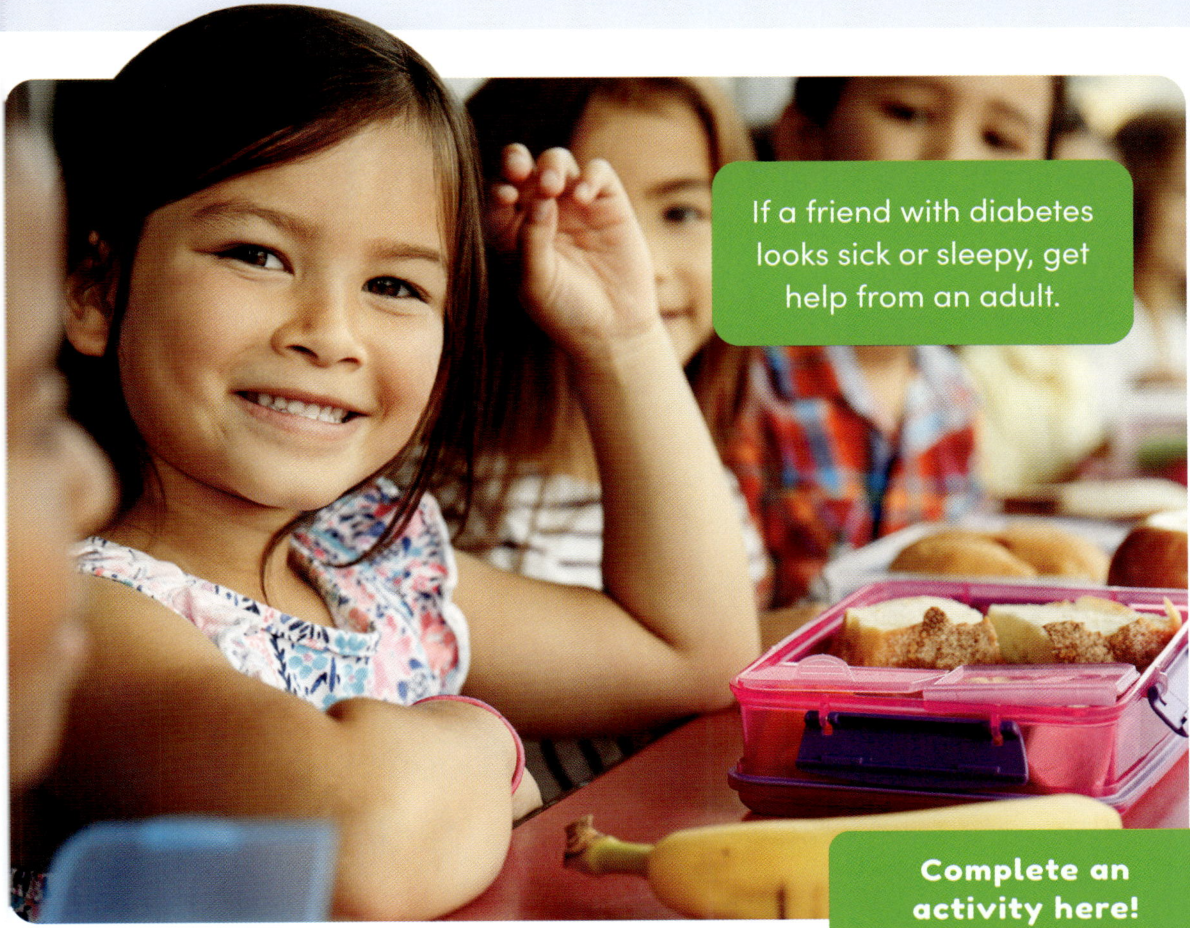

If a friend with diabetes looks sick or sleepy, get help from an adult.

Complete an activity here!

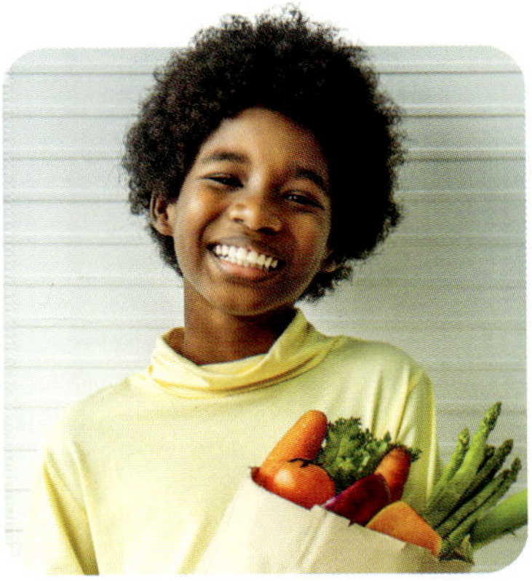

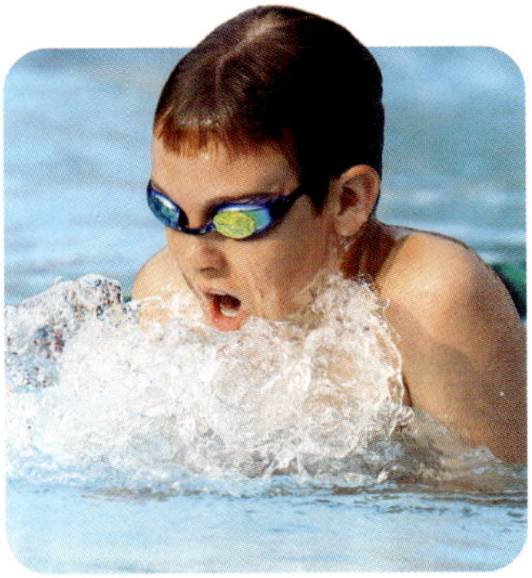

Making Connections

Text-to-Self

Do you or any of your friends have diabetes? What is having diabetes like for you or them?

Text-to-Text

Have you read any other books about people with health needs? How were those needs similar to or different from diabetes?

Text-to-World

Science has created many tools to help people with diabetes. Can you imagine any other tools that would be helpful to people with diabetes? Get creative and draw your ideas.

Glossary

automatic – moving or acting by itself.

blood sugar – the amount of glucose in the blood. It is measured as milligrams per 100 milliliters.

hormone – a chemical messenger that helps regulate activities in the body.

insulin – a hormone from the pancreas that controls the body's use of sugars. It is also a medicine used to treat diabetes.

irritable – easily bothered or angered.

Index

Online Resources

popbooksonline.com

Thanks for reading this Cody Koala book!

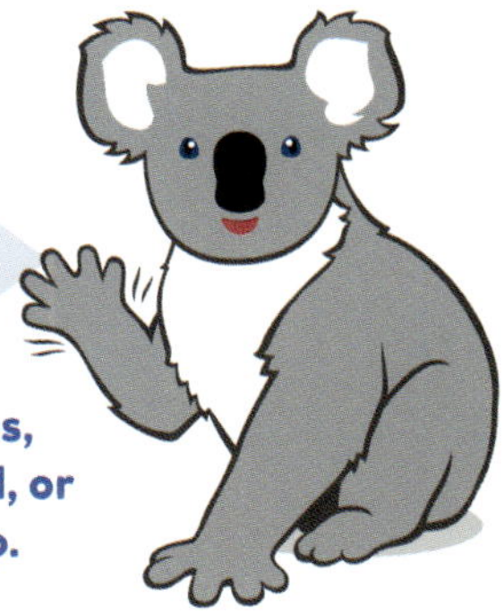

This book is filled with videos, puzzles, games, and more! Scan the QR codes* while you read, or visit the website below to make this book pop.

popbooksonline.com/diabetes

*Scanning QR codes requires a web-enabled smart device with a QR code reader app and a camera.